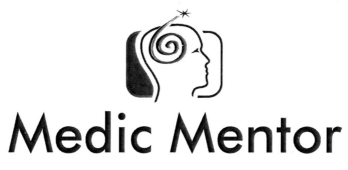

Medic Mentor
Motivating Medical Minds

> ### Medic Mentor's
> # Making it into Medicine
> ## UCAS lecture workbook

Need more help? Medic Mentor is here to support you!

Medic Mentor is a UK-wide network of approaching 1000 doctors and medical students. We understand how challenging and confusing the UCAS application process is because we have all been through it. We provide comprehensive support for the following areas:

1. *Insight into medicine conferences*

2. *Interactive lectures on competitive UCAS application*

3. *Comprehensive wider medical reading workshops*

4. *One-to-one 'Personal Statement Tutoring'*

5. *UCKAT/BMAT lectures, mock exams and structured feedback*

6. *Interview skills theory, mock interviews and structured feedback*

7. *All-inclusive Summer Schools*

8. *Institutional Bespoke Courses*

9. *10 books tackling each aspect of applying to medicine*

10. *Continuing support via our Mentor Helpline*

Find out more at www.medicmentor.co.uk

The MASTERCLASS Guide

The MASTERCLASS guide is inspired by the MASTERCLASS courses. It is a comprehensive overview of all of the topics that are taught to the MASTERCLASS students, in the years leading up to their medical school applications.

This includes the basic knowledge that students must know in order to demonstrate an insight into medicine. The guide covers the structure of the NHS, medical training, ethical principles and landmarks in Medicine and Surgery. The Guide includes notes on how to develop key skills, such as leadership, team-work, presentation, teaching and written communication. It contains guidance on study skills, time management and medical 'buzzwords', that students are expected to be familiar with. It also contains useful information about how to speak to patients and make the most of work experience.

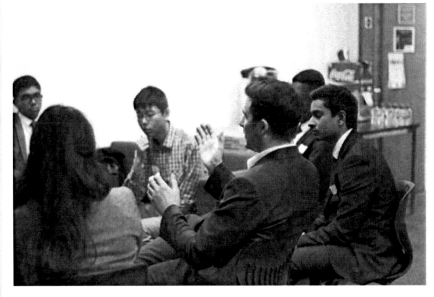

Free for MASTERCLASS Students!

For more information on how to become a MASTERCLASS student please visit www.medicmentor.co.uk

Medic Mentor®
Motivating Medical Minds

Medic Mentor's Masterclass™

The official text

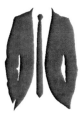

UK Medical School Applications

Dhakshana Sivayoganathan

Iain Kennedy

Ciaran Kennedy

Two Other Essential Guides

Each guide addresses important aspects of the UCAS application

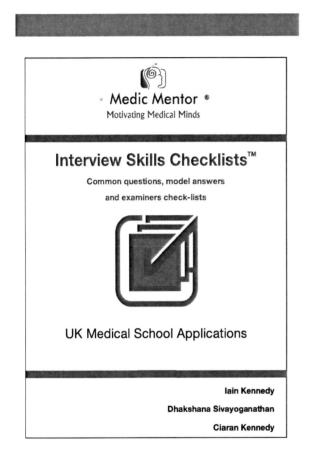

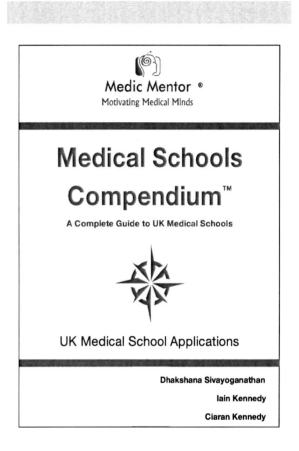

Interview Skills Checklist

This highly anticipated guide contains common interview questions asked by universities, with model answers, space to construct your own answers, followed by a mark scheme for each question. This is a fantastic guide for practicing interview questions, as it allows the student to be tested whilst the interviewer uses the mark scheme to score their answers! It also includes chapters on the structure of Medical School Interviews and the way in which these are scored.

Medical Schools Compendium

The Compendium addresses one of the most crucial and overlooked aspects of the application process: choosing the right universities to apply to. This important decision can affect the outcome of your application. This guide gives a clear breakdown of all of the UK medical schools and the facts; including competition ratios and course structures – in one place! The compendium also explains the significance of your university choices and strategies to narrow down your decision from 35 schools to just 4!

Available to order now at www.medicmentor.co.uk

THE TRUTH ABOUT A MEDICAL CAREER

What do Doctors do?

Teach, learn and practise medicine...

It is helpful to know what you are letting yourself in for before you decide to pursue a career in medicine. This can be problematic, as what doctors do on a daily basis varies from one specialty to another. Daily routine also depends upon your level of training. A basic outline of senior doctors' roles, is listed below:

Consultant Physician	Consultant Surgeon	General Practitioners (GPs)
<ul><li>Ward rounds</li><li>Clinics</li><li>Teaching junior colleagues</li><li>Administrative work</li><li>Research</li><li>Attending conferences</li><li>Multidisciplinary Team Meetings (MDTs)</li></ul>	<ul><li>As per consultant physicians</li><li>**Theatre lists**</li></ul>	<ul><li>Surgery appointments</li><li>Home visits</li><li>Administrative tasks</li><li>Teaching juniors</li><li>Research</li><li>Can attend MDTs</li><li>'Special Interests' accreditation (GPwSI's can even perform minor procedures)</li></ul>

Individually, these roles may not look demanding. Doctors however, are usually required to fulfil most of the above roles every week. A heavy and varied workload in a medical career is a common challenge. Variety is also a major draw to the career – you are unlikely to have time or cause to feel under-stimulated. Before you reach these levels however, you must first complete medical school   and your junior doctor years. Here is a basic breakdown of your expected roles:

What do Junior Doctors do?	What do medical students do?
<ul><li>Ward jobs – bloods, cannulae etc.</li><li>Review sick patients</li><li>Assist or run ward rounds</li><li>Supervised clinics</li><li>Assist in theatre</li><li>Home visits (GP trainees)</li><li>MDTs</li><li>Liaise with other health professionals</li><li>Attend courses and conferences</li><li>Research</li><li>Teach medical students</li><li>Sit Royal College exams</li></ul>	<ul><li>Exams: OSCEs, anatomy spot tests, written exams, clinical placements and coursework</li><li>Electives: a period of work experience which is often abroad</li><li>Research</li><li>Prizes</li><li>Fundraise</li><li>Societies</li><li>Extracurricular pursuits and career interest development</li><li>(Have fun and learn to be independent)</li></ul>

How diverse is a medical career?

Here is a list of some of the interesting career paths you can take as a doctor. This list goes beyond the basic roles and clinical responsibilities as described above:

Medicine – a rich and varied career

- **Author:** e.g. books or research articles
- **Manager:** e.g. Chief Executive of a hospital/Trust
- **Work for Pharmaceutical companies** e.g. develop and run clinical trials
- **Inventor:** e.g. design new surgical instruments
- **Philanthropy and social enterprise:** e.g. central committee member of a charity
- **Business:** e.g. private practice, GP practices or other types of companies
- **International work:** e.g. hands on work and training in developing countries, research
- **World Health Organisation, Government work,** or **Non-governmental organisations (NGOs)**
- **Sports Medicine** e.g. doctor for a sports team
- **Media:** e.g. medical journalist
- **Armed Forces:** e.g. trauma surgery/filed medicine
- **Court Presentation:** e.g. Pathology/Forensics

What qualities do you need to do these things?

Write a list of skills that you think might be transferrable to each of these jobs.
'Transferrable skill' development should be evident at interview, and in your personal statement

The biggest challenges for doctors

Listed below are common hurdles you may face, as you progress though a medical career

Medicine – a challenging career
<ul><li>**Multitasking** without making mistakes</li><li>**Prioritising** a demanding workload</li><li>You will be working **more hours per week** than the average person</li><li>It is **physically demanding** – some of us walk upwards of 10km per day</li><li>It is **emotionally taxing** – test yourself during your pre-medical work experience</li><li>You must be able to **communicate with patients** in difficult circumstances</li><li>**Paperwork, paperwork and more paperwork!**</li><li>**Cost** – including professional registration, postgraduate exams and courses</li><li>**Reducing number of posts** – leading to competition and the fact that you may have to move to an undesirable/unexpected location, to get the job you want</li><li>**Contracts** – changing terms and conditions may lead to some doctors being paid more than others.</li></ul>

How long does it take to become a doctor?

Medical training varies depending upon which route you take (including gap years). Below is a breakdown of multiple ways to become a doctor:

5 years	6 years	7 Years	8 years	9 years
Standard 5-year undergraduate medical degree	Foundation/ access course + 5-year undergraduate medicine degree	*3-year BSc/BA + 4-year post-grad medicine short course*	5-year *undergraduate dental degree* + *3-year post-grad super short course*	4-year integrated MSc/MA or Scottish BSc/BA then 5-year undergraduate medicine
	Undergraduate medicine at Oxbridge, Edinburgh, Imperial, UCL,	*Foundation Year + 6-year undergraduate course (with an intercalated degree)*	3-year undergraduate medicine course with 3-year intercalated PhD	3-year BSC/BA then 6-year undergraduate course (with intercalated MSc)
	5-year undergraduate medicine with intercalated BSc/BA or MSC/MA (after year 2, 3 or 4)			

* The St Andrews course involves 3 years of study in St Andrews itself to achieve a BSc (Hons) in Medicine. This is followed by a further 3 years at another medical institution (Aberdeen, Dundee, Edinburgh, Glasgow, Manchester, Barts). Students enter at the 3rd year of undergraduate medicine, upon completion of the St Andrews BSc (Hons).

Which medical school should I choose?

Read me later...

Medical school courses have been separated into three main types. Traditional, PBL and Integrated. Firstly, there are the traditional courses that tend to take a more subject-based approach to content. For example, separate teaching for anatomy, biochemistry, ethics etc. These courses also have a clear distinction between the pre-clinical and clinical years. The first 2-3 years would typically be spent studying basic medical sciences, including anatomy with full-body dissection. Then the latter (clinical) years would be spent in a medical setting, interacting with patients. This has been the basic formula for studying medicine for the past several hundred years. Recently, there has been a surge in the development of problem based learning (PBL) courses, which are at the opposite end of the spectrum. These courses have moved away from didactic, lecture-based teaching, to focus more upon clinical problems. There is an emphasis upon group work and self-directed learning. Notably, these courses often advocate early patient contact.

Most recently, the concept of an integrated course has been introduced to the undergraduate medical curriculum. This type of course mixes classical subject-based or didactic teaching with aspects of PBL, and early patient contact. Teaching 'subjects' has also evolved here into teaching 'body systems'. This is where basic science subjects (e.g. biochemistry, physiology and anatomy), are taught in the context of entire organ systems (e.g. Cardiovascular system), and the patient as a whole. Integrated curricula are a logical development of medical teaching for the 21st century. The difficulties arise when you are trying to choose medical schools to apply to, and they all tell you that they have an integrated curriculum.

In practice, all medical school curricula exist upon a spectrum – from traditional to PBL. It is difficult to find a wholly traditional course. St. Andrews is one example, physically separating the first 3 years into a pre-clinical BSc (Hons) degree. Here you are taught basic science subjects as you'd expect, but you will also find 'case-based learning' (CBL) too. This arguably makes it an integrated course. CBL is also just another name for 'problem based learning'. You can see that we have a similarly confusing issue; in addition to all marketing themselves as integrated but having slightly different curricula, medical schools also apply similar teaching methods under different names. You will also find CBL in other universities such as Keele and Cardiff. The trick is to look deeper into the actual teaching methods and see the fundamental similarities, and differences. Then work out which you prefer and can live with for 5+ years.

If you choose to attend one of the early pioneers of PBL such as Glasgow, Liverpool and Manchester, you might find fewer lectures and a lot more self-directed study. This tends to favour organised students, who like space to learn in their own way, but who also work well in groups. It is quite different from secondary school and takes a lot of responsibility and planning on your part. Traditional courses however, tend to have more rigid teaching time-tables with more time spent at university in lectures or seminars. You will find this teaching style to be similar to secondary school but on a larger scale. Many institutions now put all lecture material on virtual learning environments, which is helpful as most examination questions are based upon what you are taught here. Some describe this method of teaching as, 'spoon-feeding', as you are provided with the majority of information you need without having to look very far.

You should research individual medical school curricula and ideally speak to current medical students and teaching staff. Medic Mentor is a great resource for student contacts; you can find many Mentors who have recent experience of both applying to and studying at medical schools across the UK. In particular, you should look at varying approaches to clinical skills and anatomy teaching. These are also useful talking points at interview, to demonstrate your commitment to a particular institution. It also shows that you have done your research and have made an informed decision to study medicine at a particular university. Just imagine being asked the question, 'why did you apply to this medical school?'

In UK individual medical school curricula are basically the interpretation of guidance from the medical professional regulatory body. All medical schools are duty bound by the General Medical Council (GMC), to teach common learning outcomes. How they achieve these learning outcomes is largely up to them. 'Tomorrow's Doctors' online document – read the summary before your interview – sets out the basic competencies of newly qualified doctors. This is a great guide for your interview as you will notice there are many transferrable skills that you can demonstrate, even before you get into medical school. If you can demonstrate a working knowledge of what a junior doctor should be able to do, you can demonstrate a good insight into the career. Insight into medicine is a marked component of most application processes.

Apart from impressing at interview, knowledge of teaching curricula is essential for another obvious reason. You are going to be spending a significant part of your life at medical school, so make sure you love everything about the course (and the university and the facilities and the halls and the weather etc). Your UCAS application choices may come down to individual course aspects such as full-body dissections versus pro-sections alone; or the chance to do an 18-month research project versus a 6-month project; or perhaps something really specific like the opportunity to undertake a non-clinical elective in healthcare management or medical journalism.

Specific universities and letters after your name do not matter

One important aspect of medical education in the UK is that **it does not matter what university you studied at**, when you come to apply for junior doctor jobs. What does matter is your 'decile' ranking relative to your classmates. For example, you could essentially get the same grade in your finals but be in the 1st decile in Leeds and the 3rd decile in Oxford. This will affect your ranking for junior doctor jobs, when you come to choose your Foundation Year and locations. **You also will not be judged upon your university or your degree classification** (such as MBBS or MB.ChB). Even the impact of your final 'decile' ranking can be compensated for. For example, if you apply for a junior doctor job in a less competitive area and specialty rotations, you could still get your first or second choice and be very happy. The take-home point really is to aim for the university where you will be happiest, as this is where you are likely to make the most of your experience; hopefully getting good grades and making the most of all the other opportunities that come with being a medical student.

Academia is only half of the equation.

On the subject of additional opportunities for medical students, there are various factors to consider in your application, beyond the academic curriculum. For example, whether you want to live in a big city or in the countryside, the distance away from home, and the social scene. Consider these factors and combine them with your academic priorities. University prospectuses are woefully short on extracurricular activities. This is why you should make every effort to speak to current medical students. You can do this on open days or via Medic Mentor. You could even find out when the university or medical school Freshers' Fair is and pop down to check out what is available, in terms of groups and societies. A great first place to look is the university's MedSoc webpage or facebook group. This should have details of all the current sports, cultural and extracurricular activity groups set up specially for medical students. Additionally, you could explore the student union website for even more clubs and societies.

Interactive Task: *Note down extracurricular interests you might want to pursue at medical school. Add to this list after you have visited MedSoc and student union websites, and been to open days.*

Traditional   **Problem-based learning**

Interactive Task

What are your priorities for medical school? You can include features of the campus, curriculum, city, nightlife, social scene or any extracurricular pursuits. You should also think about your personality and preferred learning styles. Essentially if you could design a medical school and a university, what would it be like? This 'blue sky thinking' exercise can be used to think of questions for medical students and admissions selectors, on open days.

Diagrams to help you choose your medical school

Below are some diagrammatic representations of the differences between the two types of medical school courses. Remember that these are examples from either end of a spectrum. Most modern (integrated) course will have aspects of each curriculum type. There will be a definite curricular 'leaning' though. This will be in terms of attitude and not just course content. Again, to get a proper 'feel' for a course, you must attend an open day and/or quiz those who currently study there.

Traditional Course Curriculum

- Full-body dissections
- Curriculum usually subject-based but may be systems-based too
- Mainly didactic teaching such as lectures and the odd seminar
- Clear distinction between (pre-clinical) science year and clinical years.
- Later patient contact
- May lack dedicated research time
- Large teaching groups and theoretically limited access to tutors – exception is Oxbridge
- Potentially less self-directed study but reading between lectures is still a requirement
- Offer intercalated degrees – often compulsory
- Similar teaching methods to high school but bigger - can be daunting

---

Modern/PBL-based Curriculum

- Pro-sections at best, possibly virtual teaching
- Curriculum will focus upon clinical context. Could be systems-based to some degree
- Students are usually arranged into smaller problem-solving study groups
- Early patient contact and early clinical focus/context
- May lack dedicated research time
- smaller teaching groups, theoretically more access to tutors and other students
- Large emphasis on self-directed learning as little to no lecture-based information
- Offer intercalated degrees – varies between institutions
- Quite different to secondary school — requires motivation and organization for self-study

---

UK Medical Curricular Slants

Traditional	PBL
☐ Aberdeen	☐ Brighton and Sussex
☐ Barts	☐ Glasgow
☐ Birmingham	☐ Hull York Medical School
☐ Bristol	☐ Keele
☐ Cambridge	☐ Lancaster
☐ Cardiff	☐ Leicester
☐ Dundee	☐ Liverpool
☐ Durham	☐ Manchester
☐ Edinburgh	☐ Exeter
☐ Imperial	☐ Plymouth (Peninsula)
☐ KCL	☐ Norwich
☐ Leeds	
☐ Newcastle	
☐ Nottingham	
☐ Oxford	
☐ Queens Belfast	
☐ Sheffield	
☐ Southampton	
☐ St Andrews	
☐ St George's	
☐ UCL	
☐ Swansea (post---grad only)	
☐ Warwick (Post-grad only)	

How long does it take to become a medical consultant?

Below is an overview of medical training from completion of undergraduate studies to consultant level:

5 yrs +
Undergraduate medicine
Various entrance options and additional degrees
Assessment via examination and core competencies

FP/AFP
RECRUITMENT STAGE – Applications to UK Foundation Programme via FPAS
Selection based upon academic criteria and situational judgment testing
Academic Foundation Programme (AFP) – similar but requires CV + interview. Assessment via workplace based assessments and e-portfolio

2 yrs
Foundation programme – 6 x 4 month rotations across FY1 and FY2 years
Provisional GMC registration prior to FY1, full GMC registration prior to FY2
Membership of Royal College of Physicians (MRCP) Part 1 examination, is usually completed before end of FY2 (but not necessarily).

CMT/ACCS
RECRUITMENT STAGE – MRCP Part 1 desirable
Core Medical Training (CMT) or Acute Care Common Stem (ACCS)
Assessment continues via e-portfolio and work place based assessment

2 yrs
6-month core medical or acute care rotations across CT1 and CT2 years
Meanwhile you will sit for MRCP Part 2 and its practical counterpart, PACES.
These make you eligible for full membership of the Royal College of Physician

ST
RECRUITMENT STAGE – MRCP Part 2 + PACES + full MRCP membership
Eligible for recruitment to specialty training (ST), application and interview. Divergence from common pathway, commitment to specialty

4-6 yrs
Specialty training is approx. 4 – 6 years (ST3+), depends upon the specialty
Assessment is knowledge – based and via workplace based assessments
Progression is based upon achievement of required competencies

Cons
Advancement to consultant after certificate of completion of training (CCT) obtained upon completion of ST pathway --- now eligible to apply for fellowship of the Royal College of Physicians (FRCP). Direct application to posts is via submission of CV, academic documents and interview

What if you want to become a surgical consultant?

Below is another flow diagram to illustrate the process:

5 yrs +
- Undergraduate medicine
- Various entrance options and additional degrees
- Assessment via examination and core competencies

FP/AFP
- RECRUITMENT STAGE – Applications to UK Foundation Programme via FPAS
- Selection based upon academic criteria and situational judgment testing
- Academic Foundation Programme (AFP) --- similar but requires CV + interview
- Assessment via workplace based assessments and e-portfolio

2 yrs
- Foundation programme – 6 x 4 month rotations across FY1 and FY2 years
- Provisional GMC registration prior to FY1, full GMC registration prior to FY2
- Membership of Royal College of Surgeons (MRCS) Part 1 examination, is often completed before end of FY2 (but not necessarily).

CST
- RECRUITMENT STAGE – MRCS Part 1 desirable
- Core Surgical Training (CST)
- Assessment continues via e-portfolio and work place based assessment

2 yrs
- 6-month core surgical rotations across CT1 and CT2 years
- During this time you will sit for MRCS Part 2.
- These will make you eligible for full membership of the Royal College of Surgeons

ST
- RECRUITMENT STAGE – MRCS Part 2 needed
- Now eligible for recruitment to specialty training (ST) or higher surgical training, via application and interview
- Divergence from a common pathway and commitment to a specialty is usually required

5-7 yrs
- Specialty/higher training is normally 5-7 years (ST3+) but it depends upon the specialty
- Assessment is knowledge-based and via workplace based assessments
- Progression is based upon achievement of required competencies

Cons.
- Advancement to consultant level requires the certificate of completion of training (CCT) --- obtained upon completion of ST pathway --- now eligible to apply for fellowship of the Royal College of Surgeons (FRCS)
- Direct application to posts is via submission of CV, academic documents and interview

What about General Practice?

Below is a basic overview of the career pathway to becoming a GP:

5 yrs +
Undergraduate medicine
Various entrance options and additional degrees
Assessment via examination and core competencies

FP/AFP
RECRUITMENT STAGE – Applications to UK Foundation Programme via FPAS (Foundation Programme Application System)
Selection based upon academic criteria and situational judgment testing
Academic Foundation Programme (AFP) – similar but requires CV + interview

2 yrs
Foundation programme – 6 x 4 month rotations across FY1 and FY2 years
Provisional GMC registration prior to FY1, full GMC registration prior to FY2

GPST
RECRUITMENT STAGE – MRCGP Part 1 desirable
GP specialty training (GPST)
Assessment continues via e-portfolio and work place based assessment

3 yrs
6-month rotations across GPST 1-3 years
During this time, you will sit for MRCGP
Clinical skills assessment (CSA) Applied knowledge test (AKT) - GPST3
You will then be eligible for full membership of the Royal College General Practitioners, and to practise as a GP

GP
RECRUITMENT STAGE – register with primary care trust or equivalent
Apply for GP posts

Someone told me about 'Run-Through' training...

The only real difference here is that 'core' and 'higher/specialty training' are combined into one. This brings about the benefit of not having to reapply at ST3 level, and as such you avoid a common bottle---neck in the medical career pathway. On the other hand, you sacrifice a general/common training pathway for earlier commitment to specialty. This is great for people who know what they would like to specialise in for example, paediatrics or ophthalmology. It is not ideal for doctors who haven not chosen a career path by the beginning of FY2 – when ST applications take place.

List of Specialties that utilise run--through training

- *Ophthalmology*
- *Paediatrics*
- *Neurosurgery*
- *Maxillofacial surgery*
- *Obstetrics and Gynaecology*
- *Clinical radiology*
- *Histopathology*
- *Public Health*
- *Medical Microbiology/Virology*
- *Community sexual and reproductive health*

Working abroad as a Doctor

A Medical degree is like a passport. With a UK medical degree, you can work in most countries without the need to sit exams. European and Commonwealth countries have traditionally based their medical school curricula on the UK. You do not need to sit an exam if you want to work anywhere in Europe. If you would like to work in Australia or New Zealand, you do not need to sit an exam after, if you have full GMC registration. If you want to emigrate prior to FY1 and after medical school, you will have to sit the AMC exams or the NZREX, respectively. If you want to work in America or Canada, you will need to sit an exam known as the USMLE.

Table of eligibility for working abroad

USA	Canada	NZ /Australia	EU countries/Commonwealth
United States Medical Licensing Examination (USMLE) **3 steps: Part 1,2 can be done as an undergraduate Part 3 must be done as a postgraduate**	Medical Council of Canada Evaluating Exam (MCCEE) **2 parts: Part 2 can only be taken after 12 months of postgraduate study**	No examination is required/eligible to work in either country, provided you have full GMC registration **You must sit the NZREX or AMC licensing exams if you plan to work in either country prior to completion of FY1**	Eligible to work in the European Economic Area countries **Beware of Language barriers** Eligible to work in work in most Commonwealth countries **Check with individual medical licensing authorities**

University and Colleges Admissions Service (UCAS)

The culmination of your hard work needs to be demonstrated on your application form; every achievement must be displayed for the admission tutors to see. For this reason, having some knowledge of the UCAS system is essential when building your application.

All applications to medical school are now done online:

1. Register your account
2. Complete the online application which has the following headings:
   a. **Personal details**
   b. **Choices:** You need to know the institution codes, campus code and course codes. These are all available on the websites and prospectuses of individual medical schools.
   c. **Education:** All secondary school/college attendance and educational qualifications achieved. This includes your AS---level grades (if you are not doing linear/reformed A-levels)
   d. **Employment:** You can add up to 5 paid jobs. Work experience and unpaid volunteering, is not applicable here.
   e. **Personal Statement:** You have 1000-4000 (including spaces) of unformatted characters for your statement. Write your draft statement on a word processing document. When you are happy with your statement, copy and paste it into the online textbox.
   f. **Reference:** Your school will automatically attach a reference to your application. However, this cannot be done until you have completed all other sections of your UCAS application.
   g. **View all details:** will give you a preview of what your application looks like.
   h. Paying the application fee is either done online or via your school.

N.B. It is advisable to get in touch with your reference tutor, early. You should explain your desire to pursue a career in medicine, and do not forget to show them a copy of your personal statement. The best reference is one that reflects and compliments your statement.

Tracking your application:

Under this section of the UCAS website, you will find the following headings:

1. **Invitations for interview:** if the admissions selectors are impressed by your written application, you will be sent an invitation for interview. This will be recorded in this section and will probably be followed up by an email and/or letter.

2. **Conditional/Unconditional offers:** most of you will be given conditional offers, which will be dependent upon your final A-level results, in addition to health and DBS* checks. Unconditional offers are given to students who have already secured their A2 grades – e.g. gap year student who reapply.

3. **Replying to offers:** you will have a choice between 'firm acceptance/insurance acceptance/decline'. There will be a deadline for your replies.

* DBS stands for Disclosure and Barring Service – this screens for convictions and other exclusions from working.

Entry Requirements:

The entry requirements for universities vary from year to year. A-levels (appropriate subjects and high predictions) are a key academic requirement. GCSEs are important, as they constitute a complete examination profile. With the advent of linear (reformed) A-levels, more emphasis is gradually being placed upon GCSEs and A-level predictions. Some institutions are refusing to consider AS-level grades at all. Always check this in the prospectus before you apply. The table on the following page is a great starting point. This should be cross-referenced with university admissions tutors, who can be contacted via phone, email and on open days.

Chemistry A-level is compulsory for most universities along with a second science subject, such as maths, biology or physics. The combination of biology and chemistry seems to be the commonest. Taking A-level biology will benefit your studies in medical school. Many students take a contrasting, non---science third subject. Studying a language or a 'humanity' (e.g. History and Geography), demonstrates diversity, which could appeal to some universities. General Studies, Critical Thinking and Citizenship subjects are excluded. Take care however, as Oxbridge stipulate three sciences, London medical school look favourably on A-level maths.

Should you take three or four A-level subjects?

Some students choose to take four subjects to A2. This may be beneficial if you can get another A (or A*). It will add to your workload however, and could bring down your other grades. Think carefully and consider the entry requirements of the universities you are applying to.

You must also check what the policy is for a fourth A-level. Some universities prefer students to take four subjects and often make offers based upon this assumption. If you are forced to drop a subject by your school, you cannot be discriminated against. You should contact the university so they know your situation, and preferably have an email trail to confirm your eligibility to apply. Please note that for some institutions, **voluntarily dropping an A-level when they prefer four subjects, can make your application less competitive.**

For the International Baccalaureate (IB): you will need a minimum of 36 out of 45 points to be considered for entry at medical school. For Scottish students, Five Highers at A-grade are usually required. Please check with individual medical schools.

The following five pages contain the (academic and non-academic) entry criteria for 2016/17 UCAS application year. Please note that these details are subjects to change and should be cross-referenced with university admissions selectors.

Medical School	A-level grades	GCSE
Aberdeen	A2 - AAA (including Chem + 1 science). 30% weighting. AS not used.	A's + B's accepted, C's in Maths & English
Barts and The London	AAA inc. Chem OR Bio + 2nd science + third subject. **50% of interview selection**	AAABBB inc Biology, Chemistry, English, Maths
Birmingham	A*AA inc Biology + Chemistry. AAAA predicted. AS not used.	Yearly threshold. Minimum B in Maths, Eng, Science. **70% weighting.**
Brighton and Sussex	AAA inc Biology and Chemistry	B or above in English and Maths
Bristol	AAA inc Chemistry + another science. **12% weighting**	5 GCSEs at grade A inc. English Language, Mathematics and 2 sciences. **8% ranking**
Cambridge	Minimum offer: A Level: A*A*A inc. Chem + 2 sciences. 3+ sciences preferred	minimum C's in English, Maths and Science
Cardiff	AAA at A2 level (normally Chemistry and Biology required)	Minimum As and Bs in sciences and English
Dundee	AAA inc Chemistry + another science.	8 GCSEs considered, biology essential, minimum Bs
Durham	Minimum AAA at A level. Subjects should include Chemistry and/or Biology.	As in sciences if that subject is lacking at A-level.
Edinburgh	AAA inc Chemistry + another science + B in AS subject (unreformed) **25% weighting**	Bio,Chem, Eng, Maths Science at B+ **25% weighting**
Exeter	A*AA-AAA, inc. Chemistry + Biology + another sciences. **Tiered by grades**	Grade C or above in English Language **Tiered by grades**
Glasgow	AAA inc. Chemistry + another science.	GCSE English B
Hull York Medical School	AAA inc. Biology + Chemistry	8 GCSE'a A*-C, inc Maths + Eng grade A
Imperial College	Minimum AAA, typical A*AA. Inc. Chemistry and/or Biology	Minimum AAABB in Bio, Chem, Eng Lang, Maths, phys
Keele University	A*AA inc Chemistry or Biology + another science	As in 5 subjects. Minimum Bs Eng Lang, Maths, Sciences
King's College London	AAA (inc Biology and Chemistry) + further B in AS	B in Eng & Maths required, if not A/AS level
Lancaster	AAAb ot A*AA. inc Chemistry + Biology at A2. Reformed A-level accounted for	9 subjects assessed. inc B in Eng, Maths + Sciences. AAA AAA BBB minimum
Leeds	AAA at A2 inc Chemistry - A* at A2 not considered	6 Bs, inc Engl, Maths and Sciences
Leicester	AAA inc Chemistry. Biology at AS if not A2. **6% weighting**	C in Eng Lang, Maths +Sciences. Ranked against peers at **44% weighting**
Liverpool	A (Chemistry); A (Biology); A (3rd A level)	6As and 3 Bs to include Maths, Eng Lang + Sciences
Manchester	AAA in Chemistry + another science	7 at C+, inc Eng Lang & Maths, sciences B+, 5 subjects A or A*
Newcastle	AAA inc Chemistry and/or Biology at A or AS level	Dual Science, Biology or Chemistry at A
Norwich	AAAb with BBBC at AS (unreformed) **33% selection for interview**	6 GCSE As inc Eng, Maths, Sciences. Top 8 grades form **33% selection for interview**
Nottingham	A in chem + bio A2; 3rd A2 grade A in another subject	As in sciences, B in English + maths. 29% weighting at second screening
Oxford	A*AA in three A-levels - inc Chem + biology + another science	not specific, number of A*'s used in shortlisting process
Plymouth University	A*AA – AAA inc Chemistry + Biology	7 C+ inc Eng Lang, Maths + Sciences
Queen's Belfast	3 As at A2 + A at AS Level inc Chem + another science	Top 9 GCSEs considered
Sheffield	AS not considered, A2 AAA inc Chem + another science. Practical element must be passed.	Minimum 6 A's. Minimum C's in core subjects
Southampton	AAA inc chemistry + biology. **100% weighting at stage 2**	7 B's or above. **100% weighting at stage 2 (+ A2 predictions)**
St Andrews	AAA inc Chem and one of Bio, Maths or Phys	Generally 8 A's or 6 A*'s to be called for interview
St George's	AAA inc Chemistry and Biology to A2	top 8 subjects at A grade. More detail on university website
University College	A*AA inc Chem + Bio with A* in either of these subjects	B in English, Maths at least. Majority of A and A* grades is advantageous

Medical School	International Baccalaureate	SQA Highers
Aberdeen	36 points - 6's in science	S5 AAAAB inc. Chem at B grade
Barts & The London	38 points - 6's in science. **50% of interview selection**	AAA highers inc Bio + Chem, AA advanced inc Bio and/or Chem. **50% of interview selection**
Birmingham	7,6,6 at Higher level (including Biology and Chemistry) with 32 points overall	AAAAA in Scottish Highers and AAB in Advanced Highers including Chemistry and Biology.
Brighton & Sussex	36 points, Bio & Chem grade 6	Minimum 2 As advanced higher inc. Bio & Chem plus 2 As at higher. Other combos possible
Bristol	36 points, 18 Higher grade 6, in Chem + another science. **12% weighting**	higher AAAAB Advanced higher AA Chem & another science. **12% weighting**
Cambridge	40-41 points, inc 3 higher level at 7,7,6	Not stated
Cardiff	36 total, 18 points higher grade 6 inc. Chem and/or Bio	Not stated
Dundee	37 points, 18 higher grade 6 inc Chem + another science	AAABB grades at SQA Higher level inc Chem+ another science
Durham	38 points min. grade 5+, Higher Chem/Bio 6+. Sciences, Maths and English	AAAAA at Higher Grade including Chemistry and/or Biology.
Edinburgh	37 points, inc Chem. 6,6,7 at Higher level. **50% weighting**	AAAAB Highers inc. Chem + 2 sciencea, Chem + Bio preferred at advanced. **15+25% weighting**
Exeter	Typical 38-36. Higher level Bio & Chem 6+ **Tiered by grades**	Not stated
Glasgow	38 points inc. Chem, bio + Maths or Phys higher. 6+ in each	AAAAA or AAAABB in S5. AB in 2 advanced highers
Hull & York	36 points inc 6,6,5 inc. Bio and Chem	Typical AAAAB in S5, AA at advanced higher
Imperial	38 points inc Bio & Chem grade 6	AAA in Advanced highers. Chem and/or Bio + another science
Keele	35 points, 6 subjects inc. Chem or Bio + another science. 6,6,6 at higher level	AAAB inc 2 Science Advanced Higherr + Chem at Higher grade B
King's	35 points, 3 Higher at 6,6,6 inc Chem and Bio	AA Advanced Highers inc Chem & Bio + AAAAB in S5
Lancaster	36 points inc Bio, Chem + another science at 6,6,6 higher level	AAAAB highers, advanced higher AA inc Bio and Chem
Leeds	35 points, 6,6,6 higher level inc Chem and 2 of Bio, Maths, Phys	AAAAB Higher inc Bio + AB at Advanced Higher inc Chem A
Leicester	36 points inc higher Chem, Bio + 3rd subject. **6% as A-level**	Not stated
Liverpool	36 points, 3 higher inc 6, 6 in Bio + Chem + 6 in another subject	AAAAB-AAAAA plus Bio (A) and Chem (A) Advanced Higher
Manchester	37 points, 7,6,6 at higher inc Chem	AAAAB in Eng Lang and a science
Newcastle	38 points, grade 6 in Chem or Bio	AAAAA at Higher including Chem and/or Bio
Norwich	36 points, 6,6,6 Higher inc Biology and Chem or Physics **33% selection for interview**	Advanced Highers AAA inc Bio + Chem/Physics + grade B Higher **33% selection for interview**
Nottingham	36 points, 6,6,6 higher inc bio and chem	A in bio + chem Advanced Highers + AAAAB Highers
Oxford	39 points, 7, 6, 6 in highers	AA (Chem + another scince) in Advanced Highers + AAAAA Highers
Plymouth	38 - 36 points inc 6 in Higher Bio + Chem	AAA Advanced higher inc Chemistry + Biology
Queen's Belfast	36 points overall, including 6,6,6 at Higher level. Higher level Chemistry and Biology .	AAABB–AAAAA Highers, inc. Chem + Bio A. AA–AAA in Advanced inc. A in Chem + another science
Sheffield	37 points inc 6s at Higher inc Chem + another science	AAAAB + Advanced Highers AA inc Chem + another science
Southampton	36 points, 18 in 3 Higher inc 6 in chem + biology **100% weighting at stage 2**	AAAA Highers inc chem & bio, + A in chem + bio Advanced Highers. **100% weighting at stage 2**
St Andrews	38 points: 3 Higher 7,6,6, inc Chemistry (7) 2nd science.	AAAAB Highers inc Chem (A) + another science. BBB Advanced Highers
St George's	36 points total. 6,6,6 at Higher + Standard inc Chem or Bio to higher level	AAA in Chem and Bio. Advanced Highers: AA inc Chemistry and/or Biology
UCL	39 points, 19 from 3 highers inc Bio + Chem, one 7, two 6, no grades below 5	3 Advanced Highers at A1,A,A inc Chem and Bio

Medical School	Personal Statement (weighting)	Admissions Test (weighting)
Aberdeen	Review, not scored, evidence of career preparation essential.	UKCAT 20%
Barts and The London	not scored, used to support interviews	UKCAT 50% selection for interview
Birmingham	Not scored. Evidence of work experience and extracurricular activities essential	UKCAT 30%
Brighton and Sussex	Reviewed prior to interview. Not scored	BMAT - weighting not indicated
Bristol	Insight into medicine; transferrable skills; extracurricular interests; volunteering. **70%**	UKCAT 10%
Cambridge	reviewed prior to interview but not scored.	BMAT - weighting not indicated
Cardiff	Motivation, medical insight, responsibility, work-life balance, self-sufficiency, caring, **reference**	UKCAT - weighting not indicated
Dundee	reviewed prior to interview but not scored.	UKCAT - weighting not indicated
Durham	Not scored but read prior to offers being made.	UKCAT - variable minimum 'cut off' Durham/Newcastle
Edinburgh	Personal qualities, career exploration, non-academic achievement. **15%**	UKCAT 20% - 15% from SJT section
Exeter	Reviewed for commitment to study medicine. Not scored or used in the interview process	UKCAT minimum threshold. GAMSAT for graduates
Glasgow	reviewed prior to interview but not scored.	UKCAT - weighting not indicated
Hull York Medical School	Not scored	UKCAT - weighting not indicated
Imperial College	Motivation, Insight, community activities, transferrable skills, extracurricular activities	BMAT - weighting not indicated
Keele University	Not assessed. Post-application roles and responsibilities form required	UKCAT - weighting not indicated
King's College London	Not scored	UKCAT
Lancaster	Not scored checked for evidence of non-academic entry requirements after BMAT ranking	BMAT - weighting not indicated
Leeds	All statements read. Motivation, insight and transferrable skills elicited. Top 1000 scored.	BMAT - weighting not indicated
Leicester	Only scored for border line cases. Motivation and personal qualities assessed	UKCAT 50%
Liverpool	Scored - caring, insight, community involvement and written communication	UKCAT (GAMSAT postgrad). Detailed staging process
Manchester	No longer used. Online non-academic information required instead.	UKCAT, minimum 'cut-off'
Newcastle	Read prior to offers but not scored	UKCAT - weighting not indicated
Norwich	Reviewed formally. **33% selection for interview**	UKCAT. Performance in each subsection reviewed.
Nottingham	Assessed with reference. Skills, achievements, insight and experiences. **41% weighting**	Combined with GCSEs for **71% total weighting**
Oxford	Not scored	BMAT - weighting not indicated
Plymouth University	Not scored	UKCAT 50%
Queen's University Belfast	Used to support interview	UKCAT - weighting not indicated
Sheffield	Not scored. Evidence of insight, achievements, volunteering addressed at interview	UKCAT - minimum 'cut-off'
Southampton	only considered if invited to selection day	UKCAT - 100% at stage 1
St Andrews	Not scored but health-related work experience required to be called for interview	UKCAT - minimum 'cut-off'
St George's	Not scored	UKCAT - minimum 'cut-off'
University College London	'average', 'below average' or 'above average'. Broad criteria assessed - see website	BMAT - weighting not indicated

Medical School	Interview Method	Work Experience
Aberdeen	Seven-station multiple mini interview	Broad work experience and volunteering counted. Form completed at interview
Barts and The London	Structured panel interview/s	non-specific. Encouraged to get healthcare and volunteering exposure
Birmingham	Multiple mini-interviews.	Healthcare involvement essential. Volunteering/patient contact preferred
Brighton and Sussex	Twenty-minute semi-structured interviews	Non-specific, should be health-related, form completed at interview
Bristol	Multiple mini-interviews.	Minimum of two weeks in a care environment. Form completed at interview.
Cambridge	Panel interview/s	Realistic insight into medicine and demonstration of transferrable skills
Cardiff	Multiple mini-interviews.	Must demonstrate knowledge of career structure
Dundee	Multiple mini-interviews.	ideally 2 weeks of clinical experience
Durham	Multiple mini-interviews.	Commitment to caring - can be accomplished in ways other than clinical work experience
Edinburgh	Only graduated normally interviewed	Reflection on experience with the diseased, disadvantaged and disabled. Various sources accepted
Exeter	Seven-station multiple mini-interviews	Not mandatory
Glasgow	Panel interviews	Clinical experience not mandatory. Must have insight into medicine, demonstration of interest
Hull York Medical School	multiple mini-interviews.	Not mandatory. Must have insight into medicine
Imperial College	Panel Interview/s	Work experience in a clinical/healthcare setting is strongly favoured
Keele University	Multiple mini-interviews.	Experience in caring roles preferred
King's College London	Multiple mini-interviews.	Experience in a health-related setting which is verified in the personal statement.
Lancaster	Multiple mini-interviews.	Not mandatory. Insight into medicine is essential. Volunteering just as valuable
Leeds	Multiple mini-interviews.	Experience in a (broadly defined) healthcare setting,
Leicester	multiple mini-interviews.	Broad experience accepted. High quality reflection in key.
Liverpool	multiple mini-interviews.	Not specific, non-academic insight required, form completed at interview.
Manchester	multiple mini-interviews.	voluntary and caring experience required. Shadowing not necessary.
Newcastle	multiple mini-interviews.	emphasis on commitment to caring
Norwich	Multiple mini-interviews.	Non-specific. Insight and transferrable skills required. Form completed at interview
Nottingham	Eight-station multiple mini-interviews.	Voluntary experience mandatory and career insight gained from some exposure to doctors.
Oxford	Multiple panel interviews at two colleges	non-specific but required for insight into medicine
Plymouth University	Panel interview/s	no specific requirements
Queen's University Belfast	Multiple mini-interviews.	not specific but volunteering and healthcare exposure encouraged
Sheffield	Multiple mini-interviews.	Focus upon learning from and reflecting upon experiences
Southampton	Assessment Centre Selection Day	Learning from working with people in healthcare settings. No formal criteria
St Andrews	Multiple mini-interviews.	Broad definition of 'health-related' experience required on statement for interview selection
St George's	Multiple mini-interviews.	Broad scope. Learning and reflection very important. References or other evidence asked for at interview
University College London	Panel interview/s	Broad scope, learning/reflection/skill development sought. 1/3 students asked for placement verification

Medical School	Number of applicants per place	Number of applicants per interview
Aberdeen	10.9	2.4
Barts and The London	7	3
Birmingham	5.4	1.7
Brighton and Sussex	14.3	3.8
Bristol	17.6	4.4
Cambridge	6	N/A
Cardiff	12	N/A
Dundee	10.2	2.7
Durham	7	2.4
Edinburgh	13	-
Exeter	14.3	3.4
Glasgow	8	3
Hull York Medical School	7.7	2
Imperial College	N/A	N/A
Keele University	N/A	N/A
King's College London	7	3
Lancaster	9	2
Leeds	N/A	N/A
Leicester	11.9	1.9
Liverpool	7.3	1.9
Manchester	6.1	2.9
Newcastle	7.9	3.6
Norwich	9.8	2.4
Nottingham	10.1	4.1
Oxford	N/A	N/A
Plymouth University	10	3
Queen's University Belfast	N/A	N/A
Sheffield	9	4
Southampton	4	2
St Andrews	N/A	N/A
St George's	7.5	2.3
University College London	6	3

Adding to your Academic Portfolio

Many students achieve high grades in their exams, and it can be hard to distinguish yourself academically. Additional academic courses/qualifications can help to boost your academic profile.

The Extended Project Qualification (EPQ)

An EPQ is an optional project that is equivalent to an AS subject. It is also possible to attain an A* grade. Please note that EPQs are not currently interchangeable with other academic criteria, they are appealing to many institutions however (as you can see below).

The EPQ can be based on any academic topic. It can be a live production (e.g. charity event), an artefact (e.g. built technology), or a dissertation. Alongside these final products, students fill in a reflective log, which assesses their progress. You will also deliver a presentation summarising your achievements. The reflective log and final product are submitted and assessed to produce an overall grade.

Universities have praised the EPQ as it develops students' experience of self-directed learning, time management and research methods. Oxford University Medical School state on their website:

"We recognise that the [EPQ] Project might provide you with an opportunity to develop research and academic skills relevant for studying Medicine. You are therefore encouraged to draw upon your experience of undertaking the project when writing your personal statement, particularly if the topic is relevant to medicine".

Brighton and Sussex Medical School (BSMS) share a similar stance to Oxford stating:

"BSMS welcomes candidates who have successfully completed an Extended Project, recognising the effort that they have expended and the valuable skills and knowledge that they will have gained".

There are a variety of areas related to medicine that can be studied. Here are just a few:

- *Medical Ethics (e.g. Informed Consent, capacity etc)*
- *Medical Law (e.g. Gillick Competence)*
- *Health Care Policy (e.g. Review of the Health & Social Care Act)*
- *Specific Disease of interest (e.g. Alzheimer's Disease)*
- *Specific treatment/medicine (e.g. Methotrexate in Rheumatoid Arthritis)*

*Use the box below to note down any ideas for an EPQs (remember to be **specific**)*

Further educational courses

Futurelearn.com have a range of medically relevant, online courses. They are run by universities and are available for free to school/college students. Some of these courses even provide certificates that may add substance to your medical application. Below are a few course examples:

- *Medicines adherence: supporting patients with their treatment* – **King's College London**
- *Good brain, bad brain: drug origins* --- **University of   Birmingham**
- *Exploring anatomy: the human abdomen* --- **University of   Leeds**

iTunes U is an application that can be downloaded on your smartphones/iPads. It contains **free** study modules produced by universities. There are many medicine---related productions available to **download, such as:**

- *Mind the Medicine Gap* – **The Open University**
- *Obesity and Diabetes* – **University of Oxford**
- *Inherited diseases* – **The Open University**

Online Learning with Medic Mentor

- Free academic network
- School societies online
- Regional mentor network
- Freely downloadable resources
- Online learning modules

Medic Mentor has launched its brand new online academic network. Signing up for a free account lets you communicate with medical students and doctors across the country. This is a great way to network and learn about both applying to and studying medicine. Join us today on wwwmedicmentor.co.uk

Medic Mentor is also working on online courses in partnership with educational institutions. Please check www.medicmentor.co.uk regularly for updates.

Make a list below of online courses or study modules that you have found:
(Check out MedicMentor.co.uk for lots of medical application modules)

Medical Admission Examinations

There are two entrance exams for undergraduate medicine; the UK Clinical Aptitude Test (UKCAT) and the Biomedical Admissions Test (BMAT). You may only need to take one of these exams, if you are applying to schools that use the same entrance exam.

UKCAT	BMAT	GAMSAT
1. University of Aberdeen	1. Brighton and Sussex Medical School (not internationals)	1. Cardiff postgraduate
2. University of Birmingham	2. Imperial College London & postgraduate applicants	2. Liverpool postgraduate
3. University of Bristol	3. Keele University (International applicants, otherwise UKCAT)	3. Nottingham (Derby) postgraduate
4. Cardiff University	4. Lancaster University	4. St Georges postgraduate
5. University of Dundee	5. University College London	5. Swansea (postgraduate)
6. University of East Anglia (Norwich)	6. University of Cambridge	
7. University of Edinburgh	7. University of Leeds	
8. University of Exeter	8. University of Oxford & Postgraduate applicants	
9. University of Glasgow		
10. Hull and York Medical School		
11. Keele University		
12. King's College London (KCL) & Postgraduate applicants		
13. University of Leicester		
14. University of Liverpool		
15. University of Manchester		
16. University of Newcastle & Postgraduate applicants		
17. University of Nottingham		
18. Plymouth University		
19. Queen Mary, University of London & Postgraduate applicants		
20. Queen's University Belfast		
21. University of Sheffield		
22. University of Southampton & Postgraduate applicants		
23. University of St Andrews		
24. St George's, University of London		
25. University of Warwick (Postgraduate only course)		

Data correct as of May 2016 – UKCAT website, BMAT website, Individual Institution websites

The United Kingdom Clinical Aptitude Test (UKCAT)

This test aims to distinguish between candidates by assessing their mental abilities, attitudes and professional behaviour. The test is performed on a computer at Pearson Vue test centres across the UK.

There are 5 sections:

- *verbal reasoning,*
- *quantitative reasoning,*
- *abstract reasoning,*
- *decision analysis*
- *situational judgment testing (SJT).*

N.B. as of 2016/17 application year, decisional analysis is being removed and universities are starting to pay more attention to the SJT. Remember to confirm with individual institutions as to how they weight, score and consider the UKCAT.

Although it is not possible to revise material for an aptitude test, there are several ways to practise and prepare for the UKCAT.

Registration for the UKCAT **opens on May 3rd** and **costs £65 if sat between the 1st July and 31st August.** After this date, the UKCAT can be **sat up until October 4th,** but will **cost £80.** If you are worried that you may be unable to fund the cost, you might be eligible for a UKCAT bursary (which will fund either part or all of the cost). The deadline for a bursary application is the 21st September.

For more details visit: www.ukcat.ac.uk
0161 855 7409 (UKCAT Helpline)

The Biomedical Admissions Test (BMAT)

This is a 2-hour written examination, comprising multiple-choice questions, short-answer questions and an essay. The BMAT takes place on November 2nd with results published November 23rd. Last date for appeals is December 2nd. The BMAT has three sections:

- *aptitude and skills*
- *scientific knowledge and applications*
- *scientific essay*

It is also possible to prepare for this exam. The scientific knowledge section is based on the national curriculum (Key stage 4), so you are not expected to know complex medical information. The BMAT registration fee is **£45** if you register for your test by the **1st October.** If you register after this date then you have to pay an **additional £32,** up to **the final deadline of 15th October.** If you want to **appeal your BMAT result**, then the cost for this is **£33.** If you are worried that you cannot afford the cost of these tests, **contact the Admission Testing Service on 01223553366.** For more details visit www.admissiontestingservice.org

Different Routes into Medicine

You can apply to four medical schools only, via UCAS. This leaves once choice as a backup. Also, you are only permitted to apply to **either** Oxford or Cambridge medical school – **not both**. Overall, there are 32 institutions that offer undergraduate medical degrees. In addition to this, there are many other 4-year 'fast track', and 6-year combined foundation/access/gateway degrees.

The Medical Degree

32 medical schools offer a standard medical qualification (i.e. bachelor of medicine and surgery). Although the degree titles come in various forms (e.g. MBBS, MB.ChB, BM), they are all equivalent and interchangeable. It does not actually matter where your degree is from, when you apply for junior doctor jobs. This is because you are ranked against your colleagues in your institution only and put into deciles (groups of 10 percent). You will then be entered to the Foundation Programme Application System (FPAS), which is a UK-wide, standadised job-application portal.

Somebody told me about 'intercalated degrees'…

An intercalated degree gives you the opportunity to study an area of interest to a higher level (i.e. Bachelors or Masters degree). You can take part in research, learn new skills and have a break from your medical studies. Intercalated degrees add an additional year to your training. They can be costly and require hard work. Consequently, only around 50% of students choose to intercalate. Be aware however, some schools (e.g. Oxbridge, London, Edinburgh, St Andrews) incorporate an intercalated degree in their curriculum, which is 6 years as standard. Nottingham Medical School gives its students a BMedSci degree, after their first three years. This looks good, takes no more time and will give you extra points in a job application. It is **not** equal to a BA/BSc however, at least when it comes to applying for foundation jobs.

4-year fast track

This is a condensed medical degree for post-graduate entry. In addition to undergraduate qualifications, some medical schools will also require you to sit the graduate medical school admission test (GAMSAT). It seems likely that this examination will eventually be replaced with the UKAT, but this is not certain yet. Below is a table of academic entry requirements for available 4-year fast-track courses. Be aware that these grades are subject to change each year and some institutions will still look at you're A-levels and GCSEs. Each year, more postgraduate entry courses seem to become available but some also close, such as the course at Keele Medical School. It's worth doing some of your own research to see whether any other courses are likely to become available, perhaps whilst you are doing an undergraduate degree or access course.

Previous academic qualification	2.2	2.1	1st
Science degree	Imperial if you also have a PhD	Barts, Bristol, Leicester, Liverpool, Oxford & Warwick	Birmingham
Non-science degree	St George's, Nottingham	Cambridge, Kings, Newcastle, Southampton, Swansea	--

N.B. Masters degrees are generally considered to be worth the equivalent of a 1st class honours degree (or slightly higher). PhD's or doctorates are considered to be higher again.

Foundation and access courses

There are three main approaches:

1) A 5-year undergraduate medical course with an addition year (zero), as a prelude to the main course. This is a 6-year, run-through foundation programme.
2) A stand-alone science foundation year with competitive access to the 5-year medical degree. Students could potentially apply to other medical schools, if they accept foundation year qualifications.
3) An access course is any degree programme that offers transfer onto a medical degree. On example is a BSc course that allows students to transfer (competitively), into the first or second year of medicine. Students who do not secure a place in medicine could potentially complete the BSc and reapply as a postgraduate applicant.

Integrated foundation courses

These courses are for students who do not have the requisite grades or the appropriate subjects, to enter undergraduate medicine. Curricula typically focus upon basic study skills, scientific essay writing and laboratory techniques, in addition to teaching basic scientific theory in relation to medicine. Some of these of these courses have restrictive entry criteria, whilst others are available to anyone. Most integrated 6-year courses will take the place of one of your four medical choices on the UCAS form. Below is a table of 6-year, run-through foundation courses and their entry requirements:

A-levels	AAA	AAB	ABB	BCC	CCC	None
Science	--	--	--	East Anglia	Southampton, Nottingham, Kings (CCCc)	Liverpool
Non-science	Dundee (20 places)	Cardiff (AABc), Bristol, Keele, Sheffield (AABb)	Manchester	East Anglia		Liverpool

For students, who perhaps have higher grades or who just missed out on the entry requirements for medicine, consider the many 'access courses- for your 5th UCAS choice. These are discussed on the following page.

Access course – a detailed example (adapted from www.bradford.ac.uk)

Access courses are more varied than foundation programmes. They range widely in their routes into medicine, competition ratios and options available if you don't make it into medicine. You should research each course individually and evaluate its benefits and drawbacks. Below is an example of the University of Bradford, Clinical Sciences programme. This was developed in conjunction with the University of Leeds School of Medicine, as a widening access course for local student. In practice, it provides multiple routes into Leeds School of Medicine, each with relatively good odds. It is therefore and excellent option for your 5th UCAS choice.

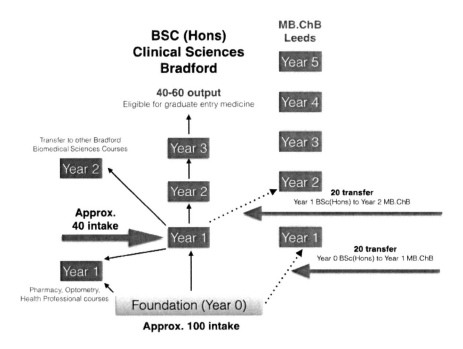

Below is a selection of foundation and access courses. None of institutions have medical school. It is worth researching universities with medical schools as they all have some form of 'access programme'. This is likely to be geographically and financially restrictive however. There are several BSc and MSc courses in some universities that also offer academically competitive transfers to medicine, without the need to fulfill geographical or socio-economic criteria.

- University of Bradford
- Carmel College
- City and Islington College
- City College Norwich
- Lambeth College
- Manchester College of Arts and Technology
- Sussex Downs College
- Thames Valley University
- College of West Anglia

Studying medicine abroad

Competition for a place at medical school in the UK is at an all---time high. There are a number of international medical courses that are largely taught in English. The compromise here is that they are expensive, require payment up front (not eligible for student loans), and they require you to emigrate. In Prague for example, you are also required to learn the local language for your clinical placements. You may also find the cultural shift daunting.   It is important to identify courses that allow you to practice in the UK when you graduate (if that is your intention). There are a few that are not directly compatible with the UK foundation programme and may require an extra year of study, periods of unpaid shadowing work or additional examinations. Two good examples of international medical courses that allow you to work in the UK following graduation are listed below:

St Georges University Medical School, (Caribbean island of Grenada)
http://www.sgu.edu
- 5-year course
- Allows you to do your first year in the   UK
- Allows for a 2-year split foundation/internship programme in the UK and USA
- Significantly more expensive than UK medical   schools

First Faculty of Medicine, Charles University, Prague (The Czech Republic)
http://www.lf1.cuni.cz/en
- 6-year course
- Allows you to enter the UK foundation programme after qualifying
- Taught in English for three years at least, but requires you to learn Czech eventually
- Similarly priced to UK medical schools but fewer options for loans and   funding

If you are interested in international medical schools, please search for individual institutions online. Every course will have a different structure. The most important thing is to check compatibility with the UK Foundation Programme.

Private Medical School

The University of Buckingham School of Medicine provides a private medical degree. Entry requirements are listed as AAB at A-level (to include chemistry). Students study a 4.5 year curriculum, based upon the University of Leicester, and qualify with an MB.ChB. Fees are £36,000 per annum – not far off the international fees at most universities. This school is not eligible for funding from Student Finance. For more information, the website is www.buckingham.ac.uk/medicine.

Making your UCAS Choices

When selecting your UCAS choices you should consider which medical schools appeal to you most and why. We have already covered teaching styles, entry requirements, course structures and competition ratios. Now you need to take a closer look at individual institutions. Attend open days and talk to students and lecturers on the course. View the university facilities beyond the medical school, (e.g. sports complex and student union). Consider that this will be the place where you spend the next 5+ years of your life – so check out the social scene and where you might be living at the very least.

Here are the key points to consider from what has been discussed so far:

- AS/A2 and GCSE requirements
- UKCAT or BMAT
- PBL, Integrated or Traditional
- Distance from home England/Scotland/Wales/N.I.
- Academic/research opportunities
- Competition ratios
- **Also** do they do interviews – Edinburgh do not have them
- Multiple mini interviews (MMI) or panel interviews (more on this later)

Use the box below to make a list of points that you want to consider when visiting a medical school. Try to break it down into social, academic and extracurricular – or create your own system.

The fifth choice

The fifth choice should be either a foundation or an access course, or another science course related to medicine (i.e. with postgraduate application in mind). Go back and review the section on foundation and access courses. Some students are still not sure if a medical degree is for them by the time they apply. To this end, a good BSc (Hons) programme would be a sensible choice, but make sure it is a subject that you could see yourself following into a career. For example, if you hate genetics or biochemistry, do not choose it as your fifth choice just because the entry requirements are lower. The same applies to the institution – you may end up staying here for the early part of your career

Work Experience

Admissions tutors are looking for quality of work experience, over quantity. Undertaking an extended work experience placement is a great opportunity to demonstrate commitment and determination to pursue a career in medicine. You do also need to show some variety with contrasting placements. The four main areas you should seek to cover with your work experience are:

1) Primary care i.e. general practice
2) Secondary care i.e. hospital
3) Community care e.g. community pharmacy, GUM, physiotherapy, hospice
4) Voluntary sector i.e. charities

The key is to start building your work experience portfolio early. It may be more manageable to complete your placements during the summer holidays. Remember to keep going with your work experience after you have submitted your UCAS application – medical schools want see evidence of commitment.

Many applications to medical school have been unsuccessful due to a lack of detail concerning work experience. To get the most out of your work experience, it is advisable to keep a reflective diary. In particular, note down any examples of situations that you learned from or might interested to speak about in your interview. You need to demonstrate that you have the qualities required to be a doctor, by using examples from your work experience.

N.B. Research *Gibb's reflective cycle* and read examples of doctors' reflections online, to help you construct your own reflective diary.

Sources of work experience:

- *Personal contacts*: Try asking family or friends, if they have any contacts in medicine whom you might be able to shadow.
- *Your GP:* call the practice and ask if it would be possible to sit in on some surgery appointments or home visits with the district nurses – you may have to go to another practice for confidentiality reasons.
- *Your local hospital*: contact your local hospital and ask to speak to the undergraduate education department.
- *Nursing Homes:* find local nursing homes on the internet and call them to see if they woul be happy for you to visit.
- *Hospices:* A great way for students who are 18+, to learn about palliative and end---of---life care.   Again, make a list using the internet and make some calls.
- *Working with children*: not only is this a rewarding and enjoyable experience but it is also a valuable learning experience. This sort of work experience is an absolute must if you are considering a career in Paediatrics. Try contacting local

© **Medic Mentor Limited 2016**

special needs schools and ask if they need any volunteers.

- *School:* your school head of sixth form or careers advisor might have a list of useful contacts who have been helpful in the past, or even well---connected alumni.
- ***Do not forget paid work:*** you can apply for weekend jobs at your local pharmacist, as a healthcare assistant, as a telephone counsellor for groups like the Samaritans or childline, or an administrative assistant for GPs.

International work

Volunteering or working abroad is great way to gain experiences relevant to a career in medicine. Some countries may have less restrictive rules on hospital volunteering and you may get to observe some tropical surgery. There are also opportunities to learn new languages and to network with new people. The important thing is not just doing a placement abroad, but what you can get out of it. With this in mind, consider a **before, during and after** approach to your international work placement.

Things to do **before** you go on your international placement:

1. Organise a placement that is aligned with your interests e.g. building orphanages in Africa
2. Consider writing a report on your experiences
3. See if you can get involved with a charity or fundraise to help pay for your trip
4. Make sure that you have a good

camera Things to do **during** your

international placement:

1. Make lots of friends and enjoy yourself
2. Take a lot of photos and videos
3. Look out for interesting topics to read about and discuss in your interview
4. Keep a reflective journal or an online

blog Things to do **after** your international

placement:

1. Write an article or make a presentation about your experience.
2. Present your work in your school if possible – especially if your UCAS referee is your class teacher. They can write about your achievements in your reference
3. If you are really ambitious, you might want to submit your article to the student BMJ or student newspaper

Charity

A large part of being a doctor is the desire to help people. The easiest and most obvious way to demonstrate this in your statement/interview, is to participate in charitable projects.

Examples of charities that school students can get involved with:

Kenyan Orphan Project (KOP): www.KOPafrica.org
KOP was formed by 3 medical students from Nottingham University. They fundraise to support vulnerable children through their health education projects in Kisumu, Kenya.

Medecins Sans Frontieres (Doctors without borders): www.msf.org.uk
Are always looking for volunteers to help fundraise. They have internships and recruit office volunteers for their London---based office, to help with administration and communications.

CV Building

Nothing beats content and formatting when it comes to putting together a CV. If you have a lot to write about then you have already won half of the battle. All you need to master after this is formatting. We still use CVs a lot in Medicine, although a lot of job applications are done online. You should always have a CV when you attend interviews, write personal statements, apply for work experience or sometimes, prizes.

CVs can be either 2-4 page summaries, or full length CVs, which can be 5-6 pages long.

Interactive task: All CVs should have the headings listed below. For each of these headings make a bullet point list of what you have achieved so far. This will help you assess the spread of your achievements and highlight stronger and weaker areas.

Education and Qualifications

Awards, Grants and Prizes

Research Experience

Presentations

Attendance at Conferences and Courses

Publications

Teaching and Mentoring

Enterprise and Innovation

Community Involvement

Other Interests

Career Intention

Referees

If you **are** lacking content in any particular area of your CV, now is the time to start filling in the gaps! The next few sections will show you how.

Personal Statements

Approaching the personal statement can seem like a daunting task. You have only 4000 characters (including spaces), to convince the admissions selectors that you are worthy of a place at medical school. In theory writing a persuasive statement comes down to knowing what to say and how to say it. Your statement has to convey one core message: that you have what it takes to pursue a career in medicine.

In practice there is a list of topics that you should aim to cover in your statement. There is also a range of ways to turn these topics into convincing arguments. Most of you will have had plenty of experiences to draw upon, when you come to write your statement. If you take a systematic approach, this can guide you in terms of what to include and where. The structure of your statement can be viewed on two levels:

1) Firstly, the **superstructure**, including the number and order of the paragraphs and the basic topics they include.
2) Second, is individual **paragraph structure** and how to organise specific points.

Statement Superstructure

It is a good idea to start planning for your statement on a word document. There is a personal statement mind---map and worksheet available for free on the UCAS website. These are not specific   to medicine but may be of use in the initial planning stages:

www.ucas.com/sites/default/files/personal--statement-- full--size_0.pdf www.ucas.com/sites/default/files/personal- --statement--worksheet.pdf

You can start with separating the statement plan into three sections:

- *The introductory paragraph,*
- *The body of the text,*
- *The concluding paragraph.*

In the first paragraph, you should answer the question, **'why (you believe) is medicine for you'** or **'why you decided to pursue a career in medicine.'**

In the body of the text you should you should:

--- Demonstrate an understanding of what a career in medicine involves
--- Demonstrate an understanding of medicine as a caring profession
--- Demonstrate your suitability to practise medicine

- o This is where you talk about your experiences and relate them to specific skills and attributes, which you see as desirable in the practice of medicine
- o For skills and attributes think: responsibility, empathy, communication, team working skills, organisation and motivation, evidence of acadaemia, creativity and social and cultural awareness (not an exhaustive list).
- o Try to link an experience or two, with one or two of these attributes, in a single paragraph – do not forget to include a link to where these skills can be applied in medicine.
- o You should also include a paragraph on extracurricular achievements, your interests outside medicine, and how you would deal with a stressful career like medicine.

In the last paragraph you should have:

--- A very brief summary of your insight into a career in medicine
--- A very brief summary of your suitability to pursue a career in medicine
--- Re-iterate your motivations to pursue a career in medicine
--- Have enough space left to write, 'thank you for considering my application.'
- o It is courteous and subtly tells the reader your statement is well formatted and concise, as you can spare the 30+ characters just to say thank you.

Paragraph Structure

Introduction

The introductory paragraph is your chance for you to show a bit of flare, as it has the ability to catch the interest of the reader. It must be succinct and to the point, but it must also appear sincere. You have one implied question to answer – why medicine? In this paragraph you need: some background and context; specific interests and insights; and some evidence of how developing these led you (logically) to pursue a career in medicine. For example:

'I first experienced healthcare through school biology: fascinated by disease processes like atherosclerosis, medical shadowing helped me observe how disease affects people and its management. Doctors' knowledge impressed me, and I decided to pursue a career in medicine.'

What did you like/not like about this paragraph? What would you change?

The body

In the **statement superstructure** section above you get an idea of what to include here, but how do you turn that into an actual paragraph? The trick is to have a logical system for making points. This way you are unlikely to miss out important statements. An example of a logical system is, **'Point, Evidence, Explanation'** or **PEE.**

Example 1: Cover all your bases with a logical system

*'I believe I will make a good doctor because I have good team---working and communication skills **(Point).** I demonstrated these when I took part in a team assent to Everest Base Camp in Year 11 **(Evidence).** I was responsible for organising my teammates into buddy pairs, monitoring their hydration and looking for signs of altitude sickness. I communicated this information to our lead teacher and the team medic. I feel that the communication and organisational skills I utilised here are highly applicable to a career in medicine, in particular when communicating patient observations and trends to senior doctors on ward rounds **(Explanation).***

A more comprehensive system is the **Gibbs' Reflective Cycle (Gibbs 1988).** This involves the following stages:

1) **Description/Action** – what you did
2) **Feelings** – how it felt/how you coped
3) **Evaluation** – what was good and what was bad
4) **Analysis** – understanding or significance of actions
5) **Conclusion** – what was done well, what could have been done better
6) **Action plan** – how can it be improved for next time **(and make explicit links to how you can apply your skills to studying or practicing medicine in future)**

Example 2: Gibbs-style.

'*During a team assent to Everest Base Camp, I was responsible for monitoring regular hydration and signs of altitude sickness in my teammates [Description]. I felt that I coped well with the responsibility [Feelings] and I was able to effectively alert my teachers to a teammate who became unwell quickly [Evaluation]. As a result of my timely actions, my teammate received medical attention [Analysis]. I felt that there was more we could have done to prevent the onset of altitude sickness [Conclusion]. I suggested that we take breaks at regular intervals, even if nobody was feeling unwell. [Action plan] This allowed everyone to acclimatise slowly, and nobody else showed any signs of altitude sickness for the remainder of the assent.*'

This example has shown how you utilised/demonstrated a multitude of skills e.g. communication, team work, taking responsibility, working under pressure, taking initiative, reflective practice and making action plans. It is however, missing the **explicit relevance to medicine**, as stated in **example 1** above. A good idea when using Gibbs or PEE to plan your paragraphs is to add an extra point: i.e. **Relevance to medicine.**

Modified paragraph systems:

Gibbs (Modified)
1) Description/Action
2) Feelings
3) Evaluation
4) Analysis
5) Conclusion
6) Action plan
7) Relevance to medicine

Point, Evidence, Explanation **(PEE)**

Becomes...

Point, Evidence, Explanation, Relevance to medicine **(PEER)**

Example 3

'I saw evidence of similar action planning in my work experience on an acute medical ward. When a junior doctor reviewed a young boy with asthma, he identified him as likely to deteriorate rapidly, due to the trend in his observations. He called his seniors, presented the case and they consequently transferred the patient to the High Dependency Unit. Good communication between doctors led to early treatment and probably prevented an asthma attack.'

It is also important to remember that listing desirable attributes of professionals you have shadowed is only half of the task. You must talk about examples of where you have developed skills essential for good medical practice. The above paragraph would be improved by some detail on how you used your communication skills effectively, as in **example 1 + 2 above**.

It is easy to write too much in this section. Try drafting a few example paragraphs, then combining some and cutting others. You will find space limited but make sure you still use full sentences and good grammar. You may not have space to make a clear link to medicine in each paragraph. Instead you could use **PEE** for 2-3 paragraphs, and include several desirable attributes. You could then have one paragraph where you talk about medical work experience (using Gibbs), and link this to the attributes you mentioned in the previous paragraphs.

You also need to include couple of sentences that show how you could potentially deal with the anticipated stresses associated with undergraduate medical study. Here you should mention something that contrasts with rigorous academic study, like sport, acting or something social. It is helpful to use words like 'balance' and 'complimentary' to emphasise the point. There is no reason however why you cannot link useful skills such as teamwork and communication inherent within these examples, to medicine.

The conclusion

- A very brief summary of your insight into a career in medicine
- A very brief summary of your suitability to pursue a career in medicine
- Re-iterate and conclude why a career in medicine if for you
- Have enough space left to write, 'thank you for considering my application.'

How you finish your statement is up to you. It does however need to have a clear and lasting message, that brings the reader back full circle to why you should be given a place at their medical school.

'I have explored medicine through varied placements. I appreciate the importance of medical ethics; I have scientific writing experience, and a fascination for public health. I appreciate the importance of empathetic doctor---patient relationships in effective patient care, and I have demonstrated responsibility by working for a year in a pharmacy. I have excelled in extracurricular activities, representing my school in rugby, and effectively balancing work commitments with social activities. I have developed leadership, team working and teaching skills, and I seek to further these through a medical career. Ultimately, I feel prepared to study medicine and I would welcome the opportunity to pursue my chosen career path. Thank you for considering my application.'

Medic Mentor's list of 'buzzwords' and key phrases

Many students struggle to use correct terminology or forget to include key topics. This list of words and phrases will help jog your memory, and may be useful to include in your statement:

- Compassion
- Teaching
- Caring
- Empathy
- Work-life balance
- Organisation
- Team work
- Rapport
- Effective communication
- Audit
- Mentoring
- Cultural/ethical/language barriers
- Body language
- Responsibility
- Time management
- Leadership
- Action planning
- Realise limitations
- Compliance/Concordance
- Reflective practice
- Professionalism
- Stress outlets
- Patient safety
- Rehabilitation
- Patient-centred/holistic care
- Barriers to healthcare
- Working under pressure
- Ability to prioritise

References

Your school/college reference must meet two fundamental criteria:

1) Primarily, it must highlight your positive attributes and therein your suitability to pursue a career in medicine
2) Crucially, it must also reflect the standard, quality and tone of your personal statement

Most students will be told that, 'the school' will be providing their reference. It is advisable that you find out who your referee is exactly, and discuss the process with them. Tell them that you are applying to medicine, a competitive course, and that it is imperative that their reference complements your statement. It is worthwhile giving your referee a copy of your statement well in advance of the reference deadline. This will allow them sufficient time to dissect your statement and produce their reference. Some medical schools provide referee guidance and it is a good idea to give your referee a copy of this. Here is a link to the Edinburgh Medical School's referee guidance, which states that *"The Edinburgh Medical School does not normally interview school leaving applicants and therefore the Personal Statement and* **Reference** *are* **extremely important**':

http://www.ed.ac.uk/polopoly_fs/1.7200!/fileManager/guidelinesforreferees.pdf

If you are able to choose your referee then choose a teacher who you know will be able to provide you with a high quality reference, with plenty of specific details. It would make sense therefore to choose a teacher who you have a good relationship with and who has had extensive contact time with you. After your reference is complete it is a good idea to review the finished product yourself and/or get your parents to check over it. Not all schools will agree to this so check with your referee beforehand. You can also assist your referee by making a list of key achievements that you would like mentioning. Finally, always take care to be courteous and respectful when approaching your referee.

Medical School Interviews

So, you have made it past the first line of admissions selectors; they were impressed by your written application and now they want to know more about you. This is where the interview comes in. Medical schools differ in their approaches to interviewing candidates. Essentially they all want to know whether you match up to the person written about on your application.

These different interview styles relate to how individual medical schools interpret the skills, attitudes and knowledge required to study and practise medicine. There is also an obvious connection between the course style (e.g. traditional vs PBL), and what they might ask. The more traditional courses are likely to value academic prowess including prizes, extra A-level and GCSE subjects, and additional academic courses (e.g. EPQs). More modern and PBL-based courses usually look for students who are motivated, organised and likely to be good at self-directed learning. Interviewers may want to focus more upon, evidence of empathy and effective communication rather than academic achievements. If you apply a bit of common sense and research your chosen medical schools well, you may be able to anticipate a few of the interview questions or topics – and practice answering them beforehand. Some medical schools post online explanations and videos, of their interview styles and questioning techniques. One good example is the University of Leeds, School of Medicine:

http://medhealth.leeds.ac.uk/info/202/applying_for_the_mbchb/107/interviews/2

But what actually happens in an interview?

Most medical school interviews follow a simple formula. You arrive at a university and you are directed to a waiting room where you register with an administrator. You are then called into another room for a 15-30 minute interview with 2-4 people. This can be thought of as the traditional approach, and is still the accepted process in many institutions. There are small variations upon this theme, such as the inclusion of a medical student or perhaps a non-medical (or lay person), on the interview panel. Other small variations are listed below:

- The presence or absence of a table, different height chairs, and room size
- Occasionally there is an observer who does not speak
- There will nearly always be a clinician
- There will nearly always be a lecturer/teacher (who may also be a clinician)
- Some interview panels employ a 'good-cop-bad-cop' technique
- Some interview panels all seem to be 'bad cops'
- Some interview panels are unnervingly positive
- There is often a mix of senior and junior medics
- Some institutions may allow you to bring your achievement portfolio

Other useful points

It may sound obvious but you must remember to dress appropriately for an interview. Suit +/- tie for men, and skirt/trousers with a blouse/shirt or smart dress, appear to be the standard for men and women respectively. Have a good breakfast, get there early and go to the toilet. Take someone with you, talk to them and try not to pay too much attention to the fretting of other candidates in the waiting room. When you enter the interview room make sure you shake hands with the entire panel. Make plenty of eye contact with the interviewers and lean forwards a little bit when you speak. You can find some more tips online and in books but really you just need to be smart, polite, punctual and enthusiastic. They already want you if you have been given an interview, so try not to worry too much, and look happy – the rest will just flow.

What questions do they actually ask?

By the time you reach interview you should already have most of the material you need. Most questions are based upon you, your achievements and your personal statement – which you should know like the back of your hand. There will be some questions that are deliberately designed to test your critical thinking and situational judgment. An example is an ethical scenario question where a colleague has behaved inappropriately. You are asked what you would do in this situation. There is no clear right or wrong answer here. The important thing is that you communicate your reasoning, make a decision that is justified and stick with it. Below is a list of typical questions and topics for discussion in a traditional medical interview:

- Why do you want to be a doctor?
- Why did you apply to this university/medical   school?
- What is teamwork/leadership and can you provide any examples in you own experiences?
- Ethical scenario 1 – an inappropriate colleague. What would you do?
- Ethical scenario 2 – a Jehovah's Witness who needs a blood transfusion. What would you do?
- Tell me about your work experience
- Tell me about a science topic that interests   you
- Tell me about what you have done to find out whether a career in medicine is suitable for you

You can find plenty more sample interview questions on the internet and in books. This brings us back full circle to the, **'Point, Evidence, Explanation'** and **'Gibbs'** processes.

Have a go at applying these systems to the interview question below:

"Can you give me an example of a situation where you demonstrated effective teamwork or working under pressure?"

How did you find this question?

Sometimes interviewers actually help you to structure your answers. For example, they might prompt you to think about a similar area of medical practice, where the same 'skills' might be applicable. If they do not prompt you they may be waiting for you to make the link – in fact it looks good if you do not require a prompt here and just launch straight into a medical example. It is worthwhile taking a look at your personal statement before the interview and trying to anticipate what questions interviewers might ask, and where you have the evidence to provide an answer. Try writing down some simple interview questions, and use **PEE** or **Gibbs** to answers to answer them. You can go further by practicing these questions with friends and family – make sure you get some constructive criticisms. Recording your mock interview sessions is a great way to reflect upon your performance and improve your technique.

Sometimes the interviewers will stop and redirect you. This occasionally happens while you are halfway through an epic recounting of your 'best' piece of work experience. Do not worry if it happens to you as you may already have given them everything they need to tick their box. In this sense, being redirected may be a good thing. Just make sure you keep smiling and go with the flow of the interview. Essentially, the interviewers job is to get as much information out of you as possible in the time available.

Ethical and medico-legal questions

These are often designed to be new situations that you have not come across before. You are unlikely to have any experience to draw upon. It is advisable that you read about medical ethics prior to your interview. The Oxford University Press *"A Very Short Introduction to Medical Ethics"* is a great starting point. Online reading and other texts should supplement this. At the very least, you should be aware of the four ethical foundation principles:

1) Beneficence
2) Non-maleficence
3) Respect for autonomy
4) Respect for justice

In addition to these, it is advisable that you have a simple understanding of some important medico-legal topics. The following list includes some examples:

1) Gillick Competence
2) Mental Capacity Act
3) Human Fertilisation and Embryology Act
4) Human Tissue Act
5) Data Protection Act

Remember that a difficult ethical question is designed to test you, but not to catch you out. All you have to do is decide upon a course of action and justify it with your reasoning. This is much easier if you can draw upon ethical foundation principles. If you can provide some examples from ethical theory and/or cases you have read about, you will be a standout candidate.

The exceptions to the rule

Oxford and Cambridge and some of the other more academically orientated institutions, choose to take an individual approach to interviews. They are more likely to focus upon academic and science-based questions. These institutions also have a reputation for asking unexpected or slightly obscure questions. If you are going to apply here you need to start searching for previous interview questions wherever you can – the internet, previous candidates etc. Even if a question is outside your comfort zone or you were not expecting it, you can still follow a logical (e.g. Gibbs or PEE) approach to answering it. Treat these interviews in a similar way to the ethical scenarios discussed above. It is your thought process that they will be interested in so do not forget to explain your reasoning. Also remember to make decisions or suggest some action, then justify it. When answering a really obscure question, it is easy to forget the link to medicine. For this reason, if you *can* make the link, you will stand out.

Multiple Mini Interviews (MMIs)

These seem to be the future of medical interviews. MMIs are basically a series of mini interview stations. Each station tends to represent a desirable trait or skill for a prospective doctor; for example empathy, communication skills or problem solving. MMI often use multi---modal approaches. Some stations may require you to interact with mock patients; others may test your written skills or interpretation of medical media. MMIs are based on the objective structured clinical examinations (OSCEs), which are used to assess medical students' practical abilities. The 'tick---list' that would have been used in a 20---minute interview, has essentially been dissected and distributed throughout the MMI stations. Some candidates may prefer MMIs, as they provide a clear framework for the interview; students are encouraged focus on specific themes in each station. Others, who do well in longer interviews, may not do so well with MMIs. This is often because there is little time to develop rapport with the interviewers. You should find out what interview format your chosen medical schools utilise. Here is a list of example MMI stations:

Question: Why do you want to be a doctor?

Question: What do you know about the medical career pathway?

Question: What work experience do you have relevant to medicine?

Question: *(Ethics)* How should the NHS address health tourism?

Written station: Who do you think is the most significant figure in modern medicine?

Acting station: Your little brother has to go into hospital to have a minor operation but he is nervous – talk him through this. (N.B.: Remember to show **empathy!**)

Comprehension station: You are given an article from the Student BMJ about the summer vacation being too long for medical students. Summarise the article, weigh the pros and cons and formulate an informed opinion.

Situational judgment station: You are given example of things a General Practitioner is doing during work hours. You must state whether these are always acceptable, sometimes acceptable or never acceptable. Do not forget to justify your answers.

This is not an exhaustive list and all medical schools will take their own approach. The Internet is a great resource for past interview questions. It is also worthwhile contacting a student who has done a medical interview before, and asks them about their experiences. Be cautious however, as some students have to sign a non-disclosure contract before their interview.

Final interview advice

All universities use a weighted scoring system to rank applicants for interview. You are scored for each section of your application i.e. statement, grades, reference, BMAT/UKCAT. Once you are at the interview it is purely your performance on the day that determines whether you receive an offer. The interviewers are looking for specific things to tick boxes but they are also interested in the overall impression you give. If you leave the interviewers with the impression that you are polite, enthusiastic, motivated and competent, this may just give you the edge you need – especially if there is only one place left and it is a decision between you and another academically equal candidate.

The best way to approach the interview is just to be you. Remember what you have practiced in terms of rehearsed answers, but do not make your answers sound wrote---learned. If something new comes to you in the moment, do not be afraid to go with it once you have covered the basics. Make sure you link all of your points to the study and practice of medicine, and you will do well. Finally remember this important point:

You have been given an interview because they want you – do not give them a reason not to offer you a place!

Clearing and UCAS Extra

Clearing is the 'last chance' service to obtain a place at university for the next academic year. You are eligible for clearing if one or both of the following apply:

- You have no offers to medical school on UCAS track
- You did not achieve the grades necessary for medical school

You can start using clearing from 9am on A-level results day through the following link: Search.ucas.com

It is unlikely that you will receive a medical school place through clearing, however it is not impossible. If you did get the grades for medicine but you were not given a conditional offer, you should call the medical schools you applied to. There may be other students who were given conditional offers but did not make the grades; consequently, the medical school may not have filled all of it places. Alternatively, if you are the student who was given a conditional offer but your final A-level grades do not meet the entry criteria, you must contact the medical school as soon as possible. If you performed particularly well at interview or other aspects of your application were exemplary, you may still be eligible for your place. The bottom line is that **you do not know until you call the medical school**, so make sure you have the contact numbers.

If you have been through the clearing process and you were unable to attain a place at medical school, there are still other options available.

If you did not receive a place but you met the grade requirements, consider contacting the medical schools you applied to for feedback on why your application was unsuccessful. After this, analyse your personal statement for any weaknesses. If for example, you did not have enough work experience consider taking a medically related gap year. Ultimately, you should aim to improve your application in whatever ways possible and reapply to medical school the following year – do not lose hope!

Even if you did not attain the grade requirements, the door to medical school is still not completely closed. Scan through clearing for **Access/Foundation** courses such as the **University of Bradford's** *(Foundation Year in) Clinical Sciences (B990/B991)*. It is worthwhile applying to these courses as they may provide you with another route into medicine. These courses are likely to request that you attend a short-notice interview – this could end up being the most important interview of your application. It may be worthwhile making a list of medical school/access course telephone numbers, the night before just in case.

UCAS Extra

UCAS Extra is a free service that is available to students who have not received any of their 5 offers. Essentially, it is an early clearing process. If you do not hold any university offers you are eligible to make more applications to courses that still have spaces available. The list of courses with free spaces will be available on the UCAS website. You can only apply to one course at a time. Before you submit an application, call the admissions tutor and double check that you meet the eligibility criteria.

How Much Does a Medical Degree Cost?

The cost of a medical degree can be a cause of anxiety for both students and parents. A standard medical degree is 5 years long, which is already 2 years longer than other undergraduate degrees. If you include an intercalated year and a foundation year, it could be up to 7 years long. As of 2013, tuition fees have increased for students and now cost £9000 for each year of undergraduate study. The cost of an intercalated degree is the same as an additional year of undergraduate study: £9,000.

Living expenses:

Based on the BMA's 'First Year Medical Student Financial Survey' for 2012-2013, the average cost of living and working is as follows per   annum.

Accommodation = £4,418

Textbooks and other materials = £184

Cost of medical equipment = £100

Vaccinations = £126

Professional fees = £199

Other essential expenditure = 215

Travel to and from medical school and to placements = £684

Food and leisure = £2400

Clothes = £500

Funding opportunities:

Total per annum = 8,826 (for five years = 44,130)

Average cost over 5 years (tuition fees and living expenses combined)

= £44,130 + (4 X 9,000 = 36,000) = 80,130

(NHS funds tuition fees from years 5 onwards)

N.B. Funding for Welsh, Scottish and International students varies. Please visit Student Finance Wales or the Students Awards Agency for Scotland. International students should approach individual institutions and their own governments' education departments

© Medic Mentor Limited 2016

Student loans

Student Finance England, provide students with two types of loans: a **maintenance loan** and a **tuition fee loan**. The tuition fee loan will be paid directly to the University and cover your tuition fees – you do not have to pay these up front. The maintenance loan will vary depending upon your place of study. It is also means tested. The average non-means tested student will receive roughly **£3,821** (more for a student in London) per year. It is paid in three installments at the beginning of each term. Students who qualify for extra financial support can receive extra funding per year. This is a bursary and therefore does not need to be repaid.

Helpfully, the government has introduced an interactive student finance calculator to their website. This allows you to estimate the fee loans and maintenance loans (and bursaries) you could be eligible for. English students can access this online resource at this address: https://www.gov.uk/student-finance-calculator

NHS Funding and Bursary

The NHS pays for your tuition fees once you reach your fifth year of study. If you have intercalated, the NHS will cover both the fourth and fifth years of your medical degree – saving you **£18,000**. You may also be entitled to an NHS bursary, which will supplement your student bursary. This is means tested and will be available from your fifth year of study onwards. There is also NHS funding available to postgraduate fast-track medical students but this is currently under review. Please contact NHS Student Bursaries to review your eligibility.

University scholarships and awards

There are competitive opportunities for funding at university, in the form of scholarships. An example of this is the *'Excellence in Scholarship, Enterprise and Leaderships (EXSEL)'*, which awards
£8000 to 4–6 medical students per year.

Other grants and bursaries

There are several opportunities for grants from the universities and medical schools. In addition to these are national bursaries such as the **Wellcome Trust (£1000)** and the **Wellbeing of Women fund (£1000)**, which provide funding for elective placements. If you are doing research abroad you may be eligible to apply for funding from a royal college or a national charity.

Paid Work

It is possible to work during the weekends and holidays as a medical student, particularly during the earlier pre-clinical years. This becomes more difficult during your final two years as clinical placements exams and electives start to take up a lot of your spare time. There may also be warden positions available at your University. These involve supervising junior students and you typically receive around 40% reduction on university halls fees.

Prizes

There are numerous prizes on offer during medical school. National prizes are much more competitive but come with significant financial gains, and they look great on your CV. A useful (not exhaustive) list of national prizes can be found on the Royal Society of Medicine student website:

https://www.rsm.ac.uk/prizes-awards/students.aspx

Is the cost of a medical degree worth it?

Yes. You will not be expected to pay back your student loan until you are working and earning over £21,000 – which will be your first year as a doctor.

Doctors in the UK earn anything from £23,000 to £4 million a year.

Your gross salary as an FY1 doctor could be £30-35k
(the number you hear about around £23k will be your base salary)

Consultant hospital doctors start on £69,000 and salaried GPs earn over £65,000.

It would not be unreasonable to earn £100,000 a year as an establish consultant and a study in 2011 suggested that the average GP salary (including practice partners) was £120,000)

Your earning potential as a doctor will far outweigh the debt that you accumulate at medical school!

For Scottish Students

This following comprises a summary of Medic Mentor's research into the current higher education funding available to Scottish students. It is accurate to the best of our knowledge and contains information relevant to 2016/17 applications.

Please note that each year, government policy undergoes a process of review that usually results in minor changes to the funding process. This has yet to be completed for 2016 and as a result there may be some changes yet to be implemented before you apply to medical school.

The Student Awards Agency for Scotland (SAAS):

This is a government-appointed body that is responsible for providing funding for Scottish students in higher education study. As prospective medical students, you will all be applying for full-time study. Beyond this, the SAAS has the following additional eligibility criteria for funding applications:

1. *Your residence arrangements*

   o Generally speaking, you should have lived in Scotland for 3 years prior to the Autumn start date (i.e. 1st August, 3 years ago)
   o *'We will not treat you as being ordinarily resident in Scotland if your main purpose in coming here has been to receive full-time education and that you would have otherwise been living elsewhere'* SAAS

2. *Any previous study*

   o There is a 'second degree medicine and dentistry degree concession' available
   o It means that from your 5th year of study you can apply for 'full support' from the SAAS
   o This could be full non-repayable funds in Scotland but is likely to be a loan in other parts of the UK
   o There is also an allowance to re-sit one year and still be eligible for continued funding
   o If you do a 4-year Scottish undergraduate degree you could have a seamless transfer of funding into your first year of medicine – it being your 5th year of study.
   o If however you do a 3-year undergraduate then apply to medicine, you will have to pay for your 1st year of study unless you can arrange otherwise with the SAAS
   o Note that second medical degrees can be 4, 5 or 6 years long but this should not impact your funding from the SAAS – it would be safest to confirm all of your course details with them in advance of accepting a place however

3. *Where you study*

- o The tuition fees in Scotland are now £1820 and are eligible to be paid in full in a non-repayable bursary.
- o You are eligible to study anywhere in the UK and still apply for funding from the SAAS, provided that you meet the other criteria listed above.
- o This may be a partial bursary or in the form of a student loan as tuition fees elsewhere in the UK are generally £9000
- o You can now also receive funding for some European universities and these are listed at www.saas.gov.uk
- o Please also note that there are currently no NHS bursary schemes in place for Scottish medical students, irrespective of where you study. They do exist for dental students however.

4. *Maintenance funding*

- o In addition to the SAAS paying your tuition fees, there are also means tested maintenance loans and bursaries available.
- o The values for are listed in the table below
- o Note that if you are 25+, married or living apart from your parents; you have children or other dependents, your household income can be calculated based upon your income and not your parents'. This may make you entitled to a larger loan and perhaps a non-repayable bursary. You should consult www.saas.gov.uk for further eligibility criteria.
- o Remember the maintenance loans and bursaries are separate from the tuition fee loans which are determined by your university location.

SAAS: Maintenance loans and bursaries:

Household income	Bursary	Loan	Total
£0 to £18,999	£1,875	£5,750	£7,625
£19,000 to £23,999	£1,125	£5,750	£6,875
£24,000 to £33,999	£500	£5,750	£6,250
£34,000 and above	£0	£4,750	£4,750

Reading list and references:

More information on all of the above points can be found at www.saas.gov.uk. You may also find useful tips on www.money4medstudents.org. If you have any further questions that you have not been able to answer, please email our administrator at admin@medicmentor.org or contact us via facebook.com/medicmentor. Our team of mentors will be happy to assist you in any of your medical school based queries.

Funding for Welsh Students

Funding for Welsh students is a little complicated. Your tution fees are covered via a combination of grants and loans. You also get full fee funding from your 5th year of study

- **£9,000 per year total fee cost**
- **£45,000 for a 5 year degree**
- **Nothing to pay up front**
- **Wales: £5,100pa grant and £3,900pa loan**
- **Only loans are repaid, grants are free**
- **Same setup even of you go to an English or Scottish Uni**
- **From 5th year NHS Student Awards Wales pays 9k in full as a grant**

Your living arrangements during term-time	Maximum Maintenance Loan available
Living at the parental home	£3,590
Living away from home and studying at a university or college outside London	£4,637
Living away from home and studying at a university or college in London	£6,497
Studying overseas	£5,529

Above – maximum non-means tested loans

Below – maximum means-tested loans

Your living arrangements during term-time	Maximum Maintenance Loan available
Living at the parental home	£4,786
Living away from home and studying at a university or college outside London	£6,183
Living away from home and studying at a university or college in London	£8,662
Studying overseas	£7,372

Welsh funding more information

You will also start paying back your student loans, as soon as you qualify as a doctor. This will be a minimal part of your take-home salary and it comes out of your pay packet before tax. Do not let the cost of medical school put you off as the rewards are great when you become a doctor – and you get to make a difference to people's lives!

Visit Student Finance Wales to confirm your eligibility for funding and review your entitlement to fee and maintenance loans and bursaries. Other useful funding resources include money4medstudents.org and NHS Wales Student Awards Unit.

IMPORTANT DATES AND TIMELINE

- Mid-End of year 11: you must submit your A-level subject options. Confirmed in year 12
- Year 12: you sit your AS levels and the results of these will go onto your UCAS form. Linear A-levels result in more emphasis being put on GCSE grades and A-level predicted grades.
- Registration for UKCAT opens: Beginning of May to the third week in September. You must create an online account before you can book. Booking closes during the first week of October. You will not need to pay the registration fee until you actually book a place.
- UKCAT exams begin on the first week in July.
- UCAS applications open between late August and early September.
- BMAT registration begins on the first week in September. There is only one date that you can sit the BMAT, therefore when you register you must also pay the exam fee.
- UKCAT bursary deadline 19th September.
- Standard entry closing date for BMAT 1st October.
- UKCAT final date to sit the exam 2rd October.
- Late entry closing date for BMAT 15th October.
- UCAS deadline for medical applications 15th October.
- Offers for medical school interviews can start as early as the beginning of October to May.
- Deadline for online Supplementary Application Questionnaire (SAQ) for Cambridge applicants only 22nd October.
- First week in November – BMAT exam.
- End of November BMAT results released and sent to medical schools.
- Majority of Cambridge interviews conducted in the first 3 weeks of December (some are done earlier).
- UCAS Extra opens 25th February-2nd July.
- May – June A-level/IB assessments take place.
- Conditional offers will be released anytime from December to May.
- August – A-level exam results released and conditional offers confirmed.
- Clearing begins on the same day as results are released.

Please be advised that the above dates vary each application year!

We wish you the best of luck with your application!
For more information about future courses visit www.medicmentor.co.uk